HEALTH MATTERS

Hearing Loss

**Carol
Baldwin**

Heinemann Library
Chicago, Illinois

Designed by Patricia Stevenson
Printed and bound in the United States
by Lake Book Manufacturing

07 06 05 04 03
10 9 8 7 6 5 4 3 2 1

Library of Congress Cataloging-in-Publication Data
Baldwin, Carol, 1943–
    Hearing loss / Carol Baldwin.
        p. cm. — (Health matters)
Includes bibliographical references and index.
    Summary: Examines the causes, symptoms, and
    treatment of hearing loss.
    ISBN 1-40340-251-5
    1. Deafness—Juvenile literature. [1. Deaf.
    2. People with disabilities.] I. Title.

RF291.37 .B35 2002
617.8—dc21

2001007974

Acknowledgments
The author and publishers are grateful to the
following for permission to reproduce copyright
material:

Cover photograph by Michael Newman/Photo Edit

p. 4 Ulrike Preuss/Format; p. 5 Spencer Grant/Stock
Boston, Inc.; pp. 6, 17 Gabe Palmer/Corbis Stock
Market; p. 7 Visual Image; p. 8 Stephen
Agricola/Stock Boston, Inc.; p. 9 Stephen
Welstead/Corbis Stock Market; pp. 10, 11, 21 Peter
Lake; p. 12 Bubbles/Jennie Woodcock; p. 13 Bob
Daemmrich/Stock Boston, Inc./PictureQuest; p. 14
Phonic Ear, Inc.; p. 15 James King-Holmes/Science
Photo Library/Photo Researchers, Inc.; p. 16
Stephen McBrady/PhotoEdit/PictureQuest; p. 18
Corbis; p. 19 Bettman/Corbis; p. 20 Mary Kate
Denny/PhotoEdit; p. 22 Henryk Kaiser/Index Stock
Imagery/PictureQuest; p. 23 Ken Lax/Photo
Researchers, Inc.; p. 24 Jeff Owen/Stock Boston,
Inc./PictureQuest; p. 25 E. Dixon/Custom Medical
Stock Photo, Inc.; p. 26T Mark Terrill/AP Wide
World Photos; p. 26B Eric Gay/AP Wide World
Photos; p. 27T Ron Edmonds/AP Wide World
Photos; p. 27B AFP/Corbis

Every effort has been made to contact copyright
holders of any material reproduced in this book.
Any omissions will be rectified in subsequent
printings if notice is given to the publisher.

Some words are shown in bold, **like this.** You can find out what they
mean by looking in the glossary.

Contents

What Is Hearing Loss?

Hearing loss is a term that describes a person's inability to hear well. When someone has trouble hearing, we say that they have hearing loss. Some people may have hearing loss in only one ear. Others may have hearing loss in both ears.

There are different levels of hearing loss. Many people with hearing loss are able to hear some sounds. Some people can hear loud sounds, but not quiet sounds. Some can hear sounds that are low in pitch, like a dog growling, but not sounds that are high in pitch, like a bird singing.

Deafness is a kind of hearing loss so great that a person cannot hear spoken language. Some deaf people can hear almost nothing, even with very powerful **hearing aids.** These people are said to be **profoundly deaf.** However, very few people can hear nothing at all.

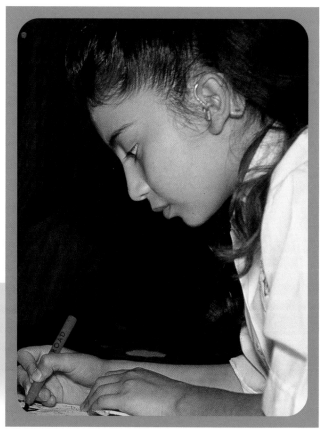

With the right kinds of help, students with hearing loss do just as well in school as anyone else.

4

Learning to speak

A major problem for children who are deaf is learning to speak. You learned to speak by imitating the sounds you heard. But because deaf children can't hear, they can't learn to peak this way. They need special training.

Children with hearing loss are able to hear a certain amount. But the sounds they hear may be very faint. They may also have constant buzzing or whistling sounds in their ears. This means that the sounds a child with hearing loss does hear may be hard for him or her to understand.

When children with hearing loss learn to speak, they usually sound different when they talk than people who don't have problems hearing. This is because the child is imitating the sounds he or she hears, which do not come through clearly. Because they are not hearing sounds accurately, they do not imitate sounds accurately.

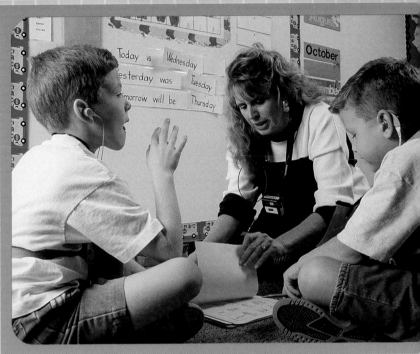

Deaf children can do just about anything that their hearing classmates can. The main difference is that they may communicate in a different way.

Sign language

Some people with hearing loss never learn to speak. Instead, they learn other ways to communicate. Many children with hearing loss learn to communicate using special **sign language** made with the hands.

5

What Causes Hearing Loss?

How you hear

To understand hearing loss, you first need to know how you hear. If you pluck a guitar string, you can see it move back and forth. These movements are called **vibrations.** Any sound, whether it's a soft whisper or a loud bang, makes the air vibrate. These vibrations are called sound waves. Sound waves travel outward in all directions from a vibrating object. You can't see sound waves, but your ears can feel their effects.

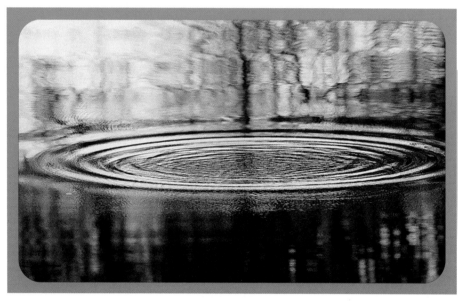

Like ripples in a pond, sound waves travel outward in all directions from the point where they started.

The outer parts of your ear collect sound waves from the air. The waves travel through your outer **ear canal.** Once sound waves travel through your ear canal, they hit your **eardrum.** Your eardrum acts like a tiny drumhead stretched over the ear canal. When sound waves hit your eardrum, it starts to vibrate. The eardrum is joined to one of three tiny bones in your middle ear. Your vibrating eardrum makes these bones vibrate too.

One of the bones in your middle ear, the stirrup, vibrates against your **cochlea.** Your cochlea is a tiny coiled tube that looks like a snail's shell. It is filled with fluid and lined with cells that have thousands of tiny hairs on their surface. The sound vibrations make the tiny hairs move. The hairs then change the sound vibrations into signals that travel along your **auditory nerve.** Your auditory nerve carries the signals to your brain. Then your brain interprets the signals and tells you what they are.

Hearing and balance

Structures in your inner ear also control your body's balance. As your body moves, fluid around tiny hair cells moves and causes signals to be sent to your brain. Your brain interprets these signals as body movements. Your brain then sends signals to your muscles to move your body to keep your balance. The hearing and balance organs are connected to each other in the inner ear. Because these organs are connected, about one in three **profoundly deaf** persons also has problems with balance.

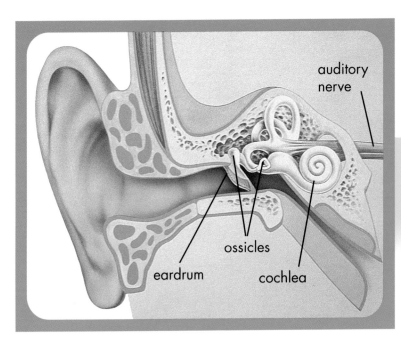

auditory nerve

ossicles

eardrum

cochlea

Inside your ear, sound vibrations are turned into signals that pass along nerves to your brain.

Types of hearing loss

There are several different kinds of hearing loss. Conductive hearing loss happens when there is a problem with part of the outer or middle ear so that sound can't reach the **cochlea.** Often this is because there is something blocking the ear passage, usually fluid in the middle ear. This kind of hearing loss can also be caused by an infection. Usually, this kind of hearing loss lasts only a short while because treatment can help.

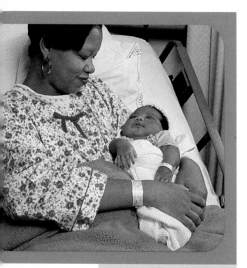

Nine out of every ten children who are born **deaf** have hearing parents.

Sensory hearing loss happens when the tiny hair cells in the cochlea are damaged or destroyed. It can affect one or both ears. Some people with this kind of hearing loss may be able to hear most sounds, but they would be muffled. Other people may be **profoundly deaf.** Sensory hearing loss is almost always permanent and sometimes gets worse. Some people have a combination of sensory and conductive hearing loss. This is called mixed hearing loss.

Neural hearing loss happens when there's a problem along the **auditory nerve** between the cochlea and the brain. Neural hearing loss can be caused when infections damage the auditory nerve. This means that messages from the ear can't reach the brain. This type of hearing loss is usually permanent.

Causes of hearing loss

There are many causes of hearing loss. Sometimes a person has hearing loss because he or she was born with parts of the ear that weren't formed correctly. Sometimes a tiny hole in the **eardrum** causes the problem. Other times, an ear **infection** or fluid in the ear causes the problem.

Sometimes hearing loss is **inherited.** You inherit all kinds of traits from your parents. Hearing loss can be inherited from one or both parents. The parents may or may not have hearing loss themselves.

Sometimes hearing loss is caused in babies when the pregnant mother catches an illness called **rubella.** Other times a child's hearing can be damaged when they get illnesses such as mumps, measles, or meningitis.

Accidents can also cause hearing loss. You can damage your ears by putting things such as fingers, swabs, or pencils in them. A serious head injury can also damage parts of the ear. That's why it's important to wear a helmet when you ride a bicycle or a skateboard.

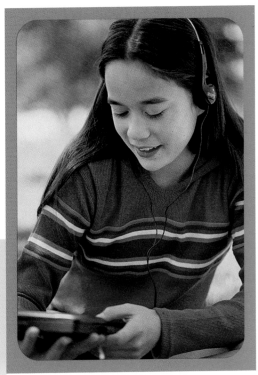

Very loud sounds can cause hearing loss. If you use a CD player with headphones, be careful not to turn the volume up too high.

9

Diagnosing Hearing Loss

Some babies are born with hearing problems. Other people are born with normal hearing and begin to have problems as they grow older. It's important for children with hearing loss to be **diagnosed** as early as possible so they can get the help they need.

Hearing tests are done when babies and young children have their regular health checkups. If a doctor thinks a child may have hearing loss, they will send the child to an **audiologist.** An audiologist is someone who is specially trained to test for hearing loss and help with problems related to hearing loss. The tests they use depend on the age of the child.

Some signs that a baby might have hearing loss:

- doesn't react to loud sounds
- doesn't smile when spoken to
- doesn't enjoy rattles or other toys that make noises
- isn't awakened by loud voices and sounds
- doesn't turn his or her head toward you when you speak

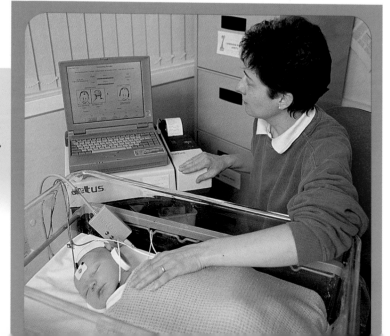

It's possible to test the hearing of babies as young as one day old. The testing does not bother the babies. In fact, some even sleep through the test.

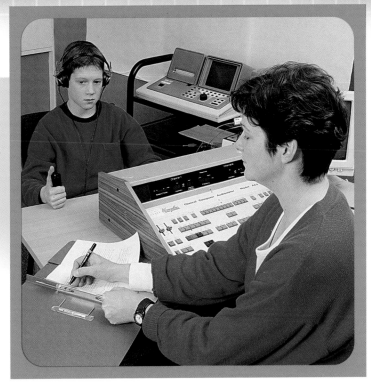

This boy is having his hearing tested. The machine beeps at different volumes and pitches so the audiologist can find out which sounds he can hear.

Testing older children

Suppose a friend goes to the doctor because he or his parents are concerned about his hearing. The doctor would first ask when your friend finds it difficult to hear. For example, is it hard for him to hear anything at all? Or does he just have trouble hearing conversations in a noisy classroom? Doctors also ask if there is anything such as a recent illness or accident that might have caused the problem. The doctor will also check your friend's ears to see if they are blocked. If not, the doctor will send your friend to an audiologist.

Different kinds of tests can be used to measure a person's hearing. The audiologist decides which tests to use. The kinds of tests the audiologist uses depend on the kind of hearing loss a person is being tested for. The results of the tests are often marked on an audiogram. This is a chart that shows what sounds a person can hear. It also shows how loud a sound has to be before they can hear it.

Treating Hearing Loss

Many people with conductive hearing loss can be treated with medicine or an operation. Most of these people will be able to hear normally again. For those who don't, **hearing aids** can help them hear better. People with sensory hearing loss can't be helped by medicine or an operation. Most of these people wear hearing aids.

Hearing aids are powered by tiny batteries. They work by using a tiny microphone to pick up sounds. The microphone changes the sounds into electrical signals. An **amplifier** in the hearing aid makes the signals louder. Then it turns the signals back into sounds and sends the sounds to the ear through a speaker. A hearing aid makes all sounds louder, not just the ones a person wants to hear.

An **audiologist** decides whether hearing aids can help a person with hearing loss. If they can, the audiologist will decide the best type of hearing aid for them. There are four basic types of hearing aids, but most children with hearing loss wear one of two types.

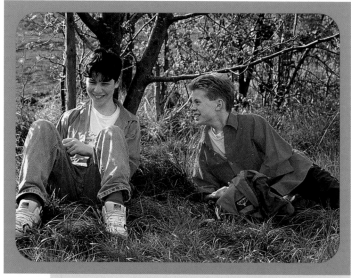

Most people find that their hearing aids work best when they are in quiet surroundings. Without background noises, such as traffic or people talking, it's easier to hear and understand what people are saying.

Types of hearing aids

Most younger children with hearing loss wear behind-the-ear (BTE) hearing aids. In this type of hearing aid, the battery, microphone, and amplifier are held in a case behind the ear. The case is connected to a plastic ear mold that fits inside the outer **ear canal.** Sound travels through the ear mold into the ear. It's important that the ear mold fits properly. If it doesn't, the wearer might get a whistling sound in his or her ears.

Older children often wear in-the-ear (ITE) hearing aids. These hearing aids are smaller and fit completely inside the outer ear. ITE aids can also hold a small coil that makes it easier to understand telephone conversations.

A few young children who are **profoundly deaf** wear body aids. This type of hearing aid is attached to a belt or pocket and is connected to the child's ear by a wire. Many children don't like these hearing aids because of their large size. They are typically used only when other types of hearing aids cannot be used.

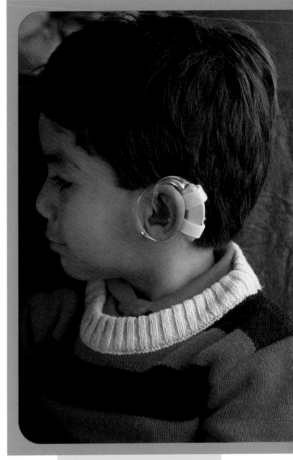

This boy is wearing a behind-the-ear hearing aid, which has two parts. One part is worn behind the ear and the other part fits inside the ear.

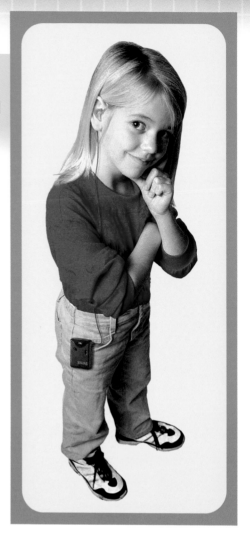

Some hearing aids can be connected directly to a television, radio, or stereo. This blocks out background noises and allows the child to hear better.

Some special **hearing aids,** called personal listening aids (PLAs), can be connected to a television set, radio, or CD player. Like a hearing aid, a PLA makes sounds louder. But unlike regular hearing aids, a PLA can make one sound, like a radio or television, louder without also making background sounds louder.

Using a computer, an **audiologist** can program some kinds of hearing aids to automatically adjust for sounds that are too loud or too soft. The wearer can change the program for different types of settings and situations. For example, a student might use one program while doing homework in a quiet room at home, and another program in a noisy classroom setting.

Getting used to any kind of hearing aid takes time. A child who has just started to wear hearing aids may have some problems. He or she will have to learn how to adjust the volume for sounds that are too loud or too soft. The child's own voice might also sound too loud to him or her at first, but he or she will get used to this over time.

Cochlear implants

Some people aren't able to hear or understand words even with hearing aids. These people may get **cochlear implants.** This involves an operation in which a very tiny device is put into a person's **cochlea.** This device takes over the job of the damaged parts of the inner ear. It sends electrical signals directly to the **auditory nerve.** Other parts of the implant are outside the body. The parts both inside and outside of the body help people with cochlear implants hear. Hearing through an implant may sound different from normal hearing, but it allows many children to learn to speak better and even talk on the telephone.

Both **deaf** children and adults get cochlear implants. Adults who lose their hearing can connect sounds made through an implant with sounds they remember. This helps them understand speech without relying on **lip-reading.** Most children who receive cochlear implants are between two and six years old. Children who receive implants at an earlier age seem to learn to speak more easily.

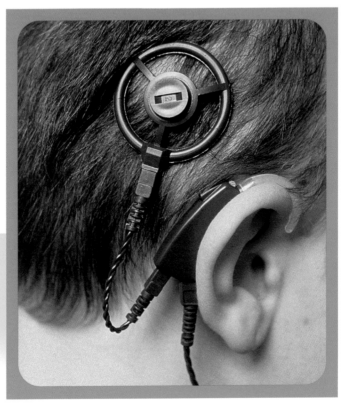

Cochlear implants can help people vary the tone of their own voices. This makes their speech easier for others to understand.

Classmates with Hearing Loss

Some **deaf** children go to special schools that are just for deaf students. Others attend special classes held in a regular school. In some schools, students with hearing loss may spend only part of their day in special classes. The rest of the time they are in classes with hearing children. Still other deaf children attend schools that are **mainstreamed.**

Some children don't like wearing their **hearing aids** in school because they may be embarrassed by them. And, their voices might sound different when they talk. These things can make them feel different, so sometimes other children may tease or pick on them. If you have a classmate who is being teased, you should tell your teacher.

Mainstreamed schools

In a mainstreamed school, all children learn together in the same classroom. Mainstreaming lets you get to know all different types of classmates. Most children with hearing loss like going to a mainstreamed school. They like being with different kinds of people, and they can make friends with other children who live near them.

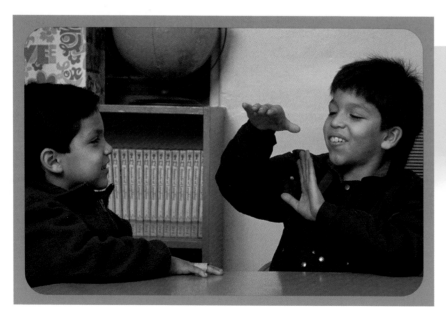

In a mainstreamed classroom, children learn that everyone has different needs, as well as different strengths.

Radio aids

Teachers who teach mainstreamed classes are trained to make sure all students learn the way that is best for them. Some classmates with hearing loss may do just fine using only hearing aids.

Other classmates need some extra help to hear what the teacher is saying. They might use an FM system or a **radio aid.** With this system, the teacher wears a special microphone. It sends what the teacher says directly to a receiver connected to your classmate's hearing aid. If you and your classmates go to a different teacher for art class, for example, your classmate can just take the microphone with him or her. Then the art teacher can use it to communicate with your classmate. You and the other students in class can also speak toward the teacher's microphone when you speak in class. That way your classmate can better hear what you are saying, too.

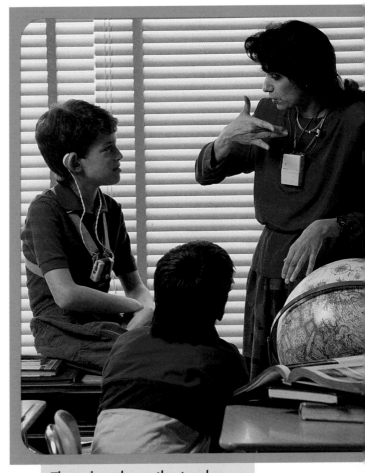

The microphone the teacher wears sends what she is saying directly to a receiver connected to the child's hearing aid. This makes it easier for the student to hear her.

Other ways of communicating

Many children with hearing loss learn different ways of communicating. Some of your classmates may **lip-read.** When they read lips, they watch the shapes that people's mouths make when they speak. People's mouths make different shapes depending on what sound they are saying. For instance, when you say the "ooo" sound, your mouth becomes round. People who lip-read can tell what someone is saying by the shapes their mouth makes when they talk.

Many **deaf** children learn a language that uses the hands, face, and upper part of the body to communicate. This is called **sign language.** In the United States, American Sign Language (ASL) is used. Other countries use different types of sign language. ASL is different from spoken English. It has its own grammar and word order.

If a classmate uses ASL, he or she may have a teacher's aide. This person uses ASL to tell your classmate what the teacher is saying.

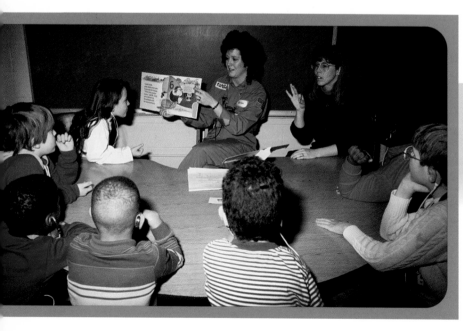

A teacher's aide who understands ASL can tell deaf students what is being said in class.

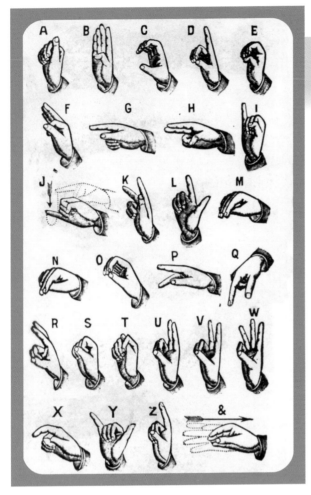

In finger spelling, each letter of the alphabet is represented by a different hand shape.

Finger spelling is another way that classmates with hearing loss may communicate. In finger spelling, different hand shapes are used for each letter of the alphabet. To communicate this way, a person moves his or her hand to spell each letter of a word in order.

Often finger spelling is used along with ASL to spell out names or unusual words. Some ASL signs use the finger letter of the first letter of the word in spoken English. For example, in ASL *group* is signed by making a horizontal circle with flat hands. *Family* is signed using the same movement, but with the *F* hand shape.

Many deaf children use a combination of ways to communicate. Some children who use ASL as their main language learn to speak as well. But these children also need to learn to read and write in English in order to do well in school.

How You Can Help

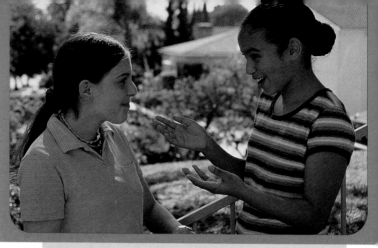

This girl makes sure she looks directly at her deaf friend while she is speaking so her friend can see her mouth as she speaks.

If someone in your school **lip-reads** or uses **hearing aids,** here are some things you can do to make communicating with him or her easier:

- Before you start talking, make sure you have your classmate's attention. Make sure he or she can see your lips as you speak.

- Face your classmate. Don't turn away while speaking.

- Pay attention to your classmate. A puzzled look may mean he or she doesn't understand what you're saying.

- Try to talk in a place that isn't too noisy.

- Don't shout. Shouting changes the way you move your mouth when you say words. This makes it hard for a lip-reader to follow. It can also make you look angry, even though you aren't.

- Speak clearly, but not slowly. Slowing down your speech may change the way you move your mouth when you say words.

- Try to talk normally. Don't forget, everyone understands part of what other people are saying by noticing their facial expressions and their body movements.

Spending time together

Here are some tips to keep in mind when spending time with a friend who has hearing loss:

◆ Plan things to do that don't depend on hearing ability. Watch a captioned television show together. Play computer or board games. Build models together or play basketball or another game outdoors.

◆ If your friend is spending the night at your home, place night-lights in the bedroom, in the hall, and in the bathroom. This way, if there's a problem during the night, you will be able to communicate with your friend because you can see each other.

◆ If your friend uses ASL or **finger spelling,** invite him or her to teach you some of those ways to communicate. Practice those skills with your friend so you can learn to communicate better.

◆ Keep a pad of paper and pencil handy in case you need them to communicate difficult words or long names.

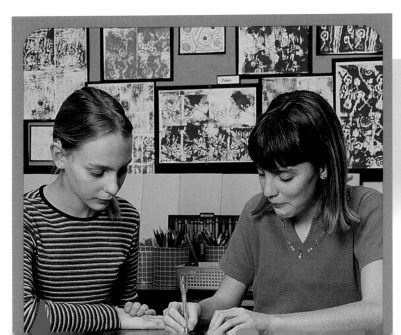

Some words may be difficult to hear or lip-read. You can use a note pad and pencil to write down anything tricky, such as an unusual name.

Visiting a Friend with Hearing Loss

Many things in your everyday life depend on hearing. These range from using the telephone to watching television. These things can be a challenge for people with hearing loss. If you visit a friend with hearing loss, you might notice that their family uses some special things to help them around the home.

You might be surprised to know that people with hearing loss use the telephone every day. Many telephones come with devices that make them easier for people with hearing loss to use. Some telephones have volume controls to make the ringer and the voice of the person on the other end of the line louder.

Other telephones have special devices in the telephone earpiece (the part that you hold to your ear) that can be used with **hearing aids.** These devices help people with hearing loss hear voices over the phone more clearly.

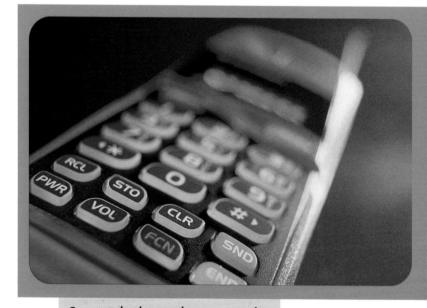

Some telephones have controls that allow the volume to be turned up. This makes it easier for people who use hearing aids to adjust the volume of a phone conversation to a level that is best for them.

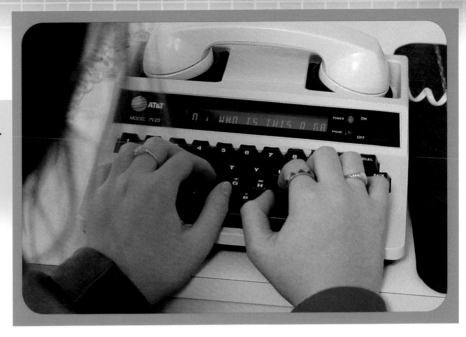

Text telephones make it easy for deaf people to communicate with friends.

Text telephones

A person who is **profoundly deaf** might use a text telephone, called a TTY. This device has a small keyboard for them to type messages on. The messages show up on a single-line screen. If the person he or she is calling also has a TTY, they can type and receive messages back and forth very quickly.

But what if a friend with hearing loss wants to call you? He or she still can, even if you don't have a TTY. All telephone companies in the United States provide a telephone relay service (TRS). TRS allows **deaf** people to communicate with people who use a regular telephone through a communications assistant (CA). Your friend dials a special phone number and types in a message to you on the other end. A CA reads the TTY message to you. Then you tell the CA what to say to your friend and the CA types your message in so your friend can read it.

Watching television

A friend who has hearing loss can enjoy watching television and movies several ways. Some children use **personal listening aids** that attach to the speaker of the television set and connect directly to their hearing aids. In addition, most television shows now have captions. Captions display, in written words, what is being said on the show. Captions appear along the bottom of the TV screen. To view captions, all you have to do is turn on the captioning feature of your television set. Captions allow both you and your friend to easily follow what is being said on the show.

At the movies

Usually subtitles are the only way to "caption" movies in theaters. Everyone in the movie theater sees subtitles. You usually only see subtitles on movies that are in a foreign language. However, a few movie theaters in the United States now have a type of captioning system for regular movies.

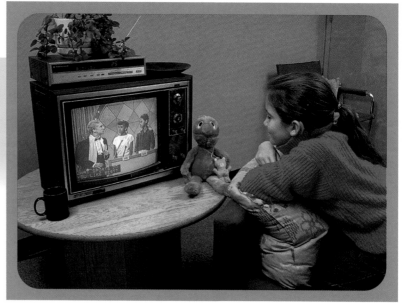

Watching a television show with the captioning on helps people with hearing loss know exactly what is being said.

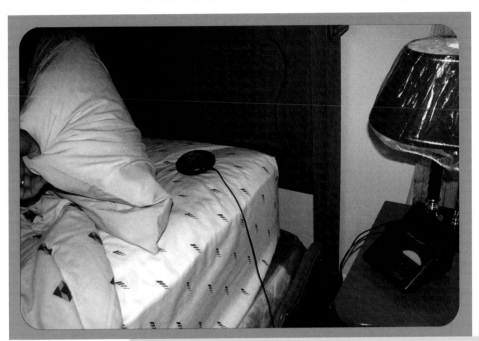

Most people who wear hearing aids take them out at night, so they can't hear a regular alarm clock. Some deaf people use special alarm clocks that have flashing lights and a vibrating pad to wake them up in the morning.

Around the house

Doorbells depend on sound. Some people with hearing loss have extra loud doorbells to help them hear the ringing. Other families have a doorbell that connects to lights in the house. The lights flash on and off when someone rings the doorbell.

A smoke alarm is another household device that usually relies on sound. Smoke alarms make loud screeching sounds when they detect smoke. This warns the family that there may be a fire. Smoke alarms can be wired to lights so they flash when the alarm goes off. Smoke alarms can even be connected to a pad under a person's pillow. The pad vibrates to wake him or her up. This allows a person with hearing loss to know when a smoke alarm goes off, even while asleep.

Hearing Loss Success Stories

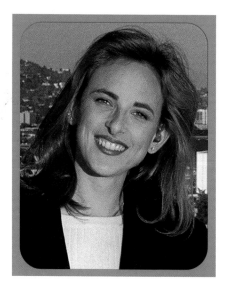

Marlee Matlin lost her hearing and became **deaf** when she was eighteen months old. Her family learned **sign language** and taught it to her as she grew up. They also talked to her while they signed. This helped her learn to **lip-read** and speak. As a child, she attended a **mainstreamed** school. Later, she began acting at Chicago's Center on Deafness. Her first movie brought her success. In 1986, at the age of 21, she won both a Golden Globe and a Best Actress Oscar. Since then, she has appeared on many TV shows.

Deaf at birth from **rubella,** Curtis Pride learned to speak as he grew up. He was always a talented athlete and played basketball and baseball in college. After college, he played for a number of baseball teams in the minor and major leagues. He has played on the New York Mets, Detroit Tigers, Atlanta Braves, and Kansas City Royals. Curtis Pride appeared on the front page of the first issue of *HiP Magazine.* This was a magazine for children who are deaf or have hearing loss.

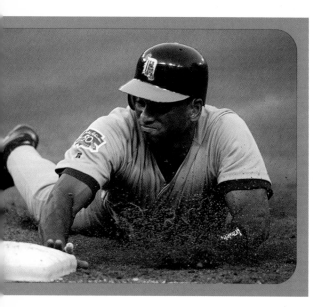

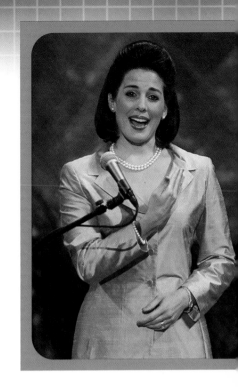

Heather Whitestone McCallum became very ill when she was eighteen months old. This left her deaf. She hears nothing in her right ear. A powerful hearing aid lets her hear some sounds in her left ear. As a child she attended a special program where deaf students learned to lip-read and speak. She also started taking ballet lessons when she was five. In 1995, her talent as a dancer helped her become the first deaf Miss America. Today she speaks to many groups about the importance of **diagnosing** hearing loss in children as early as possible.

Terence Parkin, shown below, on the left, started swimming when he was fourteen. He competed in several events in the 2000 Olympic Games and won a silver medal. What's unusual is that because he was born deaf, he has never been able to hear a race starter's signal. Instead, Terence Parkin uses a strobe light, similar to a camera flash, to signal the start of a race. He also uses **sign language** to communicate with his coach.

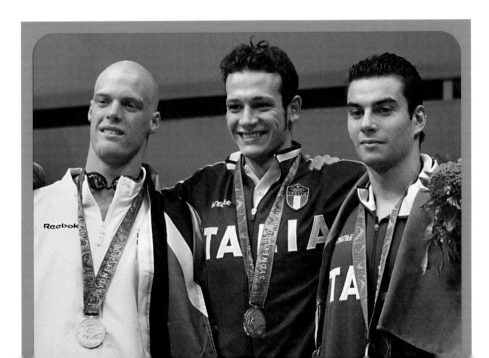

Learning More about Hearing Loss

Sign language

American Sign Language is the fourth most commonly used language in the United States. ASL uses hand shape, position, and movement to communicate. It also uses body movements and facial expressions. For example, when you ask a question, your voice usually goes up at the end of the sentence. ASL users signal a question by raising their eyebrows and making their eyes wider.

A **deaf** child with deaf parents who use ASL will learn ASL just as you learned spoken language from your parents. Hearing parents with a deaf child often choose to learn sign language along with their child. A deaf child's brothers or sisters may also learn ASL at the same time. That way, it's easier for the whole family to communicate.

To learn more about sign language, you can contact:

National Association of the Deaf (NAD)
814 Thayer Avenue
Silver Spring, MD 20910
Phone: 301-587-1788
TTY: 301-587-1789

Hearing-ear dogs

Some deaf people may have a hearing-ear dog to assist them. The dogs alert their owners to a sound by running back and forth between the owner and the sound. Examples of sounds that dogs may be trained to alert their owners to include:

◆ a siren

◆ ringing telephone

◆ fire or smoke alarms

◆ an oven timer

◆ a doorbell or knocking on a door

◆ a crying baby

The American Humane Association offers people a guide to various hearing-ear dog programs. The guide tells about each program, such as the area it serves and whether the program will train a family pet.

American Humane Association
Hearing Dog Program
9725 East Hampden Avenue
Denver, CO 80231
303-695-0811

Glossary

amplifier   device that makes sounds louder

audiologist   person who is specially trained to test for hearing loss and help with problems related to hearing loss

auditory nerve   nerve that carries information about sounds from the cochlea to the brain

cochlea   part of the inner ear that changes sound waves into signals that travel along the auditory nerve to the brain

cochlear implant   device that does the job of the cochlea; it changes sounds into electrical signals and sends them to the inner ear

deaf   having hearing loss so great that a person can't hear spoken language

diagnose   to recognize what illness or condition a person has

ear canal   tube that connects your eardrum with the outer part of your ear

eardrum   circular piece of skin that separates the outer ear from the middle ear. It passes vibrations from the air to the tiny bones in your middle ear.

finger spelling   way of communicating that uses different hand shapes to represent each letter of the alphabet. Finger spelling is often used as part of sign language.

hearing aid electronic device worn by people with hearing loss to make sounds louder

infection sickness caused by germs entering the body

inherited received from one's parents. Deafness and other characteristics can be inherited.

lip-read to understand what someone is saying by watching the shapes a person's mouth makes as he or she speaks

mainstreamed class or school that includes many different kinds of learners including gifted children and children with special needs

personal listening aid device that increases the loudness of a particular sound without increasing the loudness of background sounds

profoundly deaf level of deafness that occurs when a person can hear almost nothing, even with powerful hearing aids

radio aid device worn by a teacher that sends his or her voice directly into a child's hearing aid

rubella sickness that can cause hearing loss

sign language system of language in which people use their hands, upper parts of the body, and facial expressions to communicate

vibration small, rapid, back-and-forth motion

More Books to Read

Gordon, Melanie. *Let's Talk about Deafness*. New York: PowerKids Press, 1999.

Haughton, Emma. *Living with Deafness*. New York: Raintree Steck-Vaughn, 1999.

Landau, Elaine. *Deafness*. Brookfield, Conn.: Twenty-First Century Books, 1994.

O'Neill, Linda. *Imagine Being Deaf*. Vero Beach, Fla.: Rourke Press, 2000.

Pringle, Laurence. *Hearing*. Tarrytown, N.Y.: Marshall Cavendish, 2000.

Index